I0420086

How
To
QUICKLY
Lose
20 POUNDS
BEFORE
YOUR CHRISTMAS
PARTY

Dr. Chio Ugochukwu

Copyright © 2019 Dr. Chio Ugochukwu

All Rights Reserved. No part of this book may be reproduced in any form, or means, without the permission of the author or publisher.

Published by Bundant Enterprises

3053 Rancho Vista Blvd, H-197

Palmdale, California
ISBN-978-1077538757

Printed in the United States of America.

© Dr. Chio Ugochukwu 2019-All rights reserved

Disclaimer and Terms of Use

The author and publisher have made every effort to ensure the accuracy and completeness of the information contained in this book, we assume no responsibility for errors or omissions therein. It is solely for informational and educational purposes and should not be regarded as a substitute for professional advice. Your reliance upon information and content obtained through this book is solely at your own risk. The author and publisher assume no liability or responsibility for any adverse consequences for the use of any product, information, idea or instruction contained in this book.

© Dr. Chio Ugochukwu 2019-All rights reserved

Dedication

This book is dedicated to all those who want to quickly lose weight before an upcoming event like your Christmas party.

© Dr. Chio Ugochukwu 2019-All rights reserved

Table of Contents

© Dr. Chio Ugochukwu 2019-All rights reserved

© Dr. Chio Ugochukwu 2019-All rights reserved

"THE ABILITY

TO TAKE FOCUSED ACTION EVERYDAY

TOWARDS YOUR DAILY GOAL

IS THE DIFFERENCE BETWEEN LIVING

THE LIFESTYLE OF YOUR DREAMS AND

DREAMING OF YOUR LIFESTYLE"

DR. CHIO

8

© Dr. Chio Ugochukwu 2019-All rights reserved

Introduction

It can be quite stressful, when you want to quickly lose 20 pounds before your Christmas party and you do not have an easy and reliable way to do it. This is particularly more challenging when you have limited time and consider that the holiday season, starting from Thanksgiving to the New Year is full of social events and endless opportunities to overeat and gain weight. How can you overcome this challenge?

You can begin by finding the answers to a few critical questions. How much weight do you want to lose before your Christmas party? What steps, actions or activities will you do everyday to help you lose weight? If you truly want to lose weight and keep it off, before your Christmas party you have to be clear on why you want to lose weight,

© Dr. Chio Ugochukwu 2019-All rights reserved

how much weight you want to lose, and how you will do it. Through this book you will learn quick, simple and reliable ways and strategies that will help   you consistently lose 20 pounds before Christmas party, without getting distracted by anxiety, fear of failure while ignoring the daily distractions, criticisms and annoyances that are invariably part of your daily life!

Ask yourself what you have done in the last 24 hours to help you lose weight and keep it off. Did you take action? Did you keep to the promises you have made to yourself about eating less and smiling more often? Unless you consistently take the actions that will help you fulfill your goals, even after you have discovered why you want to lose weight, you would find yourself losing and gaining weight every week!

© Dr. Chio Ugochukwu 2019-All rights reserved

One of the secrets to fearlessly losing weight is the ability to let disappointments or unmet expectations go and continue to take consistent daily action towards your goal of relentless weight-loss. Don't dwell on your disappointments or goals that you failed to meet. Learn from them and move on.

You can easily and quickly lose 20 pounds and keep it off before your Christmas party through the compass method, which is a holistic system for relentless transformation that is based on the 7 compass profiles. It is the core method that I will share with you in this book.

© Dr. Chio Ugochukwu 2019-All rights reserved

© Dr. Chio Ugochukwu 2019-All rights reserved

Begin with a holistic –weight loss approach based on the compass profiles

Did you know that everything you do affects your weight? Begin with the end in mind. For you, the end maybe losing at least 20 pounds before your Christmas party, for others it may be 10 pounds or fifteen. Focus on your own goal, the reasons behind your goal and the benefits you will get from achieving your goal, then take action. While it is true that everything affects everything, you have to remember that intention without action leads to zero results.

Do you have an everything-related or holistic approach to weight loss? Don't assume that because you failed in your previous attempts at losing weight that you will fail again. Do you

© Dr. Chio Ugochukwu 2019-All rights reserved

have an idea of the food that typically makes you eat more than you would normally like to it? For some people it is chocolate cookies! What about you? You can find out by doing your 72-hour food audit. You can do this with your food journal or with your diary. When you do this, you will discover the driver of your weight gain and you can begin to take action immediately. If you discover that you eat too much ice cream or cake, cut it down right now. If the problem is over snacking then stop talking "one snack" for the road!

Invest in yourself. Make your weight loss holistic! Do you know how the different aspects of your daily life affect your weight? You can find this out through your compass profiles. You can also relentlessly pursue your daily weight-loss goals through the use of your compass profiles. The

© Dr. Chio Ugochukwu 2019-All rights reserved

components of the compass profile are the following:

C = Community Relationships profile.

O = Operational capacity profile.

M= Metabolic profile.

P= Physical profile.

A= Ambition profile.

S= Spiritual profile.

S = Self Knowledge profile.

How can you use these profiles to lose weight before your Christmas party? **The community relationships profile is essentially your communications profile.** The first step in using the community relationships profile is to gain a deeper understanding of yourself and others. Communicate with yourself first and write down your deepest fears and worries. What is affecting your confidence in yourself and your ability to

© Dr. Chio Ugochukwu 2019-All rights reserved

make decisions? What is holding you back from making a commitment to relentless weight loss? Is it fear of the process or fear of communication with others?

Effective communication is good because it will help you to reduce stress. The more you reduce stress the less likely you will attempt to use eating to keep stress off. Do the best you can and leave the rest. **The smallest action is better than the greatest intention**. Taking action will help you reduce stress and have more energy for all the fun things you would like to do with your life. Try to reduce complex problems to small segments that you can accomplish. Begin where you are, not where you want to be.

Ask yourself questions that will help you recognize which aspects of your relationship with

© Dr. Chio Ugochukwu 2019-All rights reserved

others could either be contributing to your weight gain or making it more difficult for you to lose weight. When you go to parties you have to eat only what you had planned to eat. If you eat to please others, you will run into trouble during the holiday season and it will be more difficult for you to lose weight and keep it off before your Christmas party!

Keep in mind that everything affects your weight loss and narrow your focus to finding out more about how you can consistently implement your daily strategy for weight loss, rather worrying about other people's smiles and approval which are usually transient.

What is your operational capacity profile? Your operational capacity is your ability to get things done, with the resources and time that you have or

© Dr. Chio Ugochukwu 2019-All rights reserved

to make adjustments, without excuses, when they are required. What is your wherewithal for achieving your goals? Do you have the money to buy the vegetables and fruits you will need to buy regularly if you want to lose weight and keep it off before your Christmas party? If you cannot afford to 5 servings of vegetables, buy two. What is your operational capacity for weight loss? Do you have a process and strategy in place that fits your worldview and personality that will help you lose weight? You have to set aside one day for fasting.

When you combine your findings from your 72-hour food audit with your **operational capacity profile,** you will know which situations and circumstances are more challenging than others. Avoid them. A weight loss journal will help you keep track of the different aspects of your weight loss journey.

© Dr. Chio Ugochukwu 2019-All rights reserved

If you are not sure of the operational capacity that will work best for you, look back at your life and find out which method of preparation and execution has worked the best for you in your most successful projects. Modify your weight loss strategy to fit that model.

Include in your project review, things like getting ready for vacations, birthday parties or getting ready for a wedding or tasks as simple as going to work on time and cleaning your house. For most people, the best way to tackle most projects is to start on time and break them down into small simple steps. For others every project is eventually done at the last minute. You cannot lose weight and keep it off through last minute approaches.

If you like to get things done at the last minute, it means you tend to procrastinate and underestimate how much time you would need to get your

© Dr. Chio Ugochukwu 2019-All rights reserved

projects completed. **You have to learn to persist and win strategically (PAWS). Remember that inadequate preparation leads to failure.** To lose weight and keep it off before your Christmas party, you have to start with a small plan and build on it slowly, in a way that suits your internal and external circumstances.

You have to use your PAWS to get your target. First, find out your weight and determine how much weight you have to lose. Do you have to lose 20 pounds, 30 pounds or 10 pounds? How much time do you have? Do you have 6 weeks, 3 months or 3 weeks? Your answers to these questions will determine how you will apply the compass method for weight loss to your situation and circumstance.

Do you know your metabolic profile? When was the last time you did your blood work? Your **metabolic profile** will include both your

© Dr. Chio Ugochukwu 2019-All rights reserved

nutritional and metabolic analysis. You can get your metabolic analysis by getting your physiological and laboratory tests done. This will help you to know if there are significant medical problems responsible for your weight struggles. Getting the right tests done with the help of a healthcare professional or your doctor will make it easy for you to know which aspect of your health profile you need to focus on improving.

When it comes to losing weight even without running tests, **your family history can help you a get a better picture of your risk factors.** If you have a family history of diabetes, hypertension, kidney disease or chronic obesity, then you have to be much more vigilant than others. It means you have factors that can either lead you to gain weight or make your weight-

© Dr. Chio Ugochukwu 2019-All rights reserved

loss more challenging. Don't forget that "more challenging" does not mean impossible!

The Physical Profile includes your weight, height, waist circumference and BMI (Body Mass Index). It also includes your heart rate and lung function. These factors are important because how healthy you are will how much vigorous exercise you can engage in. **Take action today, weigh yourself today, even if you feel you are in excellent health.**

If you want to lose weight and keep it off before your Christmas party, you have to exercise day by day. Keep it simple. Do daily mild to moderate activities like **walking**, dancing, running up and down a flight of steps, jump ropes and pushups. If you are more interested in vigorous exercise like going to the

© Dr. Chio Ugochukwu 2019-All rights reserved

gym for intense workouts or playing basketball, tennis, and baseball, you need to remember to check with your doctor to make sure that you are healthy enough to begin vigorous exercise.

One advantage of staying physically active is that it helps you burn off excessive calories that would have been converted to fat. Increased storage of excess energy in the form of fat will ultimately build up your weight and cause more health problems. In the relentless weight program you have to exercise every day!

What is your ambition profile? **The Ambition Profile** assesses your drive and motivation. What is the highest level of success you would strive for in your endeavors? Would like to lose weight and keep it off permanently or would like to lose weight for an event or an occasion

© Dr. Chio Ugochukwu 2019-All rights reserved

only? You can use the ambition profile to set **measurable goals like losing your first 10 pounds within the first 3 months of starting the *relentless weight loss* program.**

This is an important strategy because once you can confidently write down the actions and activities that helped you lose your first 10 pounds, you can build on it to lose more pounds. What is your ambition profile? Write it down as part of your own relentless weight loss program losing weight before your Christmas party.

The remaining two profiles are **Spirituality and Self Knowledge**, both of which examine your psychosocial and spiritual make up. They will help you have a **better understanding of your personality,** character and connection with God and the universe. **Knowing your personality type**

© Dr. Chio Ugochukwu 2019-All rights reserved

will give you a greater insight into how your sense of self affects your weight loss strategy.

A better understanding of your psychosocial strengths and weaknesses will help you know your limitations, when it comes to choosing pathways to better health and consistent weight loss. It will also help you to anticipate problems, challenges and pressure points.

On the spiritual side of the equation, more and more studies are beginning to show that those who meditate or are truly prayerful are better able to handle health challenges than those who do neither. Of course I realize that there are different interpretations of what it means to be spiritual and that one size does not fit all. Discover yours and embrace it! Apply it to your circumstance and desire to lose weight before the Christmas party!

© Dr. Chio Ugochukwu 2019-All rights reserved

Through the use of the 7 elements of the compass profile you will be able develop a more holistic and realistic approach that will help you to lose weight before your Christmas party!

© Dr. Chio Ugochukwu 2019-All rights reserved

Do your 72 -hour food audit and self-analysis

I already mentioned the 72- hour food audit as an important part of the compass holistic weight- loss approach? What did you eat for breakfast 3 days ago? Was it healthy? Did you snack on fruits or on chips? Do you know the patterns that dominate your relationships, activities and eating habits? Use the first 24 hours or first day of your food audit to learn as much as you can about yourself. Write down the patterns that are most prominent in your life during the past 72 hours in your weight loss journal. Identify and write down your own:

*Eating pattern

*Working pattern

© Dr. Chio Ugochukwu 2019-All rights reserved

HOW TO QUICKLY 20 POUNDS BEFORE YOUR CHRISTMAS PARTY

*Relationship pattern

*Activity pattern

*Assignment pattern

*And Meditation pattern.

*How many parties do you have to attend before your Christmas party?

Write down your meals and snacks, how much time you spend on your computer, tablet, I-pad TV, or smart phones. Do you eat and watch TV or play games with your smart phones at the same time? How do you typically deal with your emotions like anger and sadness? The more accurate and specific, you are with your answers to these questions the clearer the picture you can paint for yourself, and the easier it will be for you to know the specific adjustments you need to make

© Dr. Chio Ugochukwu 2019-All rights reserved

to your daily routine and habits to help you lose 20 pound before your Christmas party..

In the second 24 hours or second day of your 72 – hour food audit explore your metabolic profile, especially the important aspects of your family and medical history. Do you have a family or personal history of obesity –related illnesses like diabetes, high blood pressure, heart attack or stroke? Consider taking advantage of free informational health exams or blood work offered at your office or your membership clubs or insurance to get your cholesterol or metabolic profile. This will help you determine, if there is an underlying systemic illness that is making it very difficult for you lose weight, that needs to addressed.

In the third 24 hours or third day which will complete your 72 hour time frame begin to write

© Dr. Chio Ugochukwu 2019-All rights reserved

down the components of your weight-loss blueprint for the long haul. Make this your own personalized list of actions and pledges that will help you transform your health and life. This basically means taking some detailed transformative actions and applying them to your weight-loss goals.

Here is an example of a list you can make on the third day of your 72 hour time frame:

*Cut down your food portions by at least half, and make up for the difference through fruits and vegetables. This will help you feel full, while reducing your total daily calorie intake and losing weight.

*Eat your food in one location without watching TV or checking on your smart phone.

© Dr. Chio Ugochukwu 2019-All rights reserved

*Eat more grains, vegetables, fruits, milk and beans, and use oils like cranola and olive oils.

*Eat at least 10 grams of fibers daily through eating nuts like almonds and cereals like oats.

* **Stop eating processed food like bread and pizza.**

*Eat at least five servings of fruits and vegetables daily.

*Eat a delicious red apple with every meal.

*Read your nutritional facts before you buy or use your food products.

*Eat fish and skinless poultry like chicken or turkey.

*Drink low-fat milk or eat low fat yoghurt.

*Walk at least 60 minutes everyday.

© Dr. Chio Ugochukwu 2019-All rights reserved

HOW TO QUICKLY 20 POUNDS BEFORE YOUR CHRISTMAS PARTY

*Keep stress out of your relationships.

*Sleep at least six to eight hours a day.

*Cut down on unnecessary expenses.

*Call a friend today.

*Review your finances.

*Help at least one person each day.

*Meditate or say a prayer or do both.

*Form a healthy living-group of friends and family members.

*Write down your feelings and experiences.

*Repeat your blood pressure check.

*Weigh yourself every 3 days.

*Take Omega 3, vitamin D, Magnesium, lutein and vitamin C every day.

© Dr. Chio Ugochukwu 2019-All rights reserved

HOW TO QUICKLY 20 POUNDS BEFORE YOUR CHRISTMAS PARTY

*Keep your appointment with your healthcare providers.

*Keep eating healthy even after a lapse.

*Do your screening tests as recommended by your healthcare providers.

*Become familiar with your family and medical history.

*Continue to write down your emotional disruptions periodically.so that you can figure out the actions you need to diffuse or eliminate them.

*Forgive yourself and others daily.

*Keep quiet if you have nothing positive to say.

*Review and modify this list as it fits your individual needs and circumstances.

© Dr. Chio Ugochukwu 2019-All rights reserved

There you have it! These are the some of the weight-loss strategies and tips, you can develop or discover, after you have done your full 72-hour food audit. You are welcome to use them and begin to lose weight every day! Instead floating a weight-loss trial balloon, read the next chapter for more ideas and thoughts on how you can develop specific, realistic and achievable goals for quickly losing 20 pounds before your Christmas party.

© Dr. Chio Ugochukwu 2019-All rights reserved

Set specific achievable weight loss goals with realistic strategies

If you truly you want to lose weight before your Christmas party you have to set the specific actions that you will take everyday to help you lose weight. If you really want lose weight and keep it off, you have to set goals you can achieve with realistic strategies. Don't set a goal of losing 100 pounds in 1 week by going to the gym 24 hours a day for 1 week. It is neither realistic nor achievable. This is particularly the case if you have to go to work everyday and still take care of your family. **Unachievable goals lead to discouragement.**

© Dr. Chio Ugochukwu 2019-All rights reserved

Don't set the goal of never going to any parties between Thanksgiving and your Christmas party, because it is not realistic. Making your goals achievable and realistic combines the compass operational capacity profile and the ambition profile in the compass method. The good news is that **when you set an achievable goal like losing weight and keeping it off in the setting of an event, your Christmas party, your focus will narrow and you will waste less time with the resources at hand. Life will support you in every possible way and provide what you need to make fearless progress in your journey.**

Don't let your daily struggles, distractions, frustrations and criticisms prevent you from striving to live up to your full potential. You have the potential to do anything you want to do including quickly losing weight before your

© Dr. Chio Ugochukwu 2019-All rights reserved

Christmas party. **Believe in yourself!** You have all the resources you require and enough skills to live the life you intended. You can do this by believing in yourself and taking action and staying focused on achieving your daily goals one step at a time.

The key to losing weight and keeping it off during the holiday season is staying vigilant and disciplined. This means that when you feel the urge to eat ice cream or drink alcohol, you will reject it. Even though you may enjoy drinking, you have to remember, that it gives you non-nutritious calories while keeping your liver busy. You also have to refuse any offers of all the sugar-loaded enticing delights, that friends and family will invariably make to you during this time of the year. Haven't you noticed that it always seems that every time you make up your mind no to do

© Dr. Chio Ugochukwu 2019-All rights reserved

something, counter thoughts urging you to the opposite kick in. REJECT THEM!

If you truly want to relentlessly lose weight before your Christmas party, you have to learn to have a specific optimistic focus for the hours that make up your day. If you do not do this, you will not have an anchor to help you stay committed to effective implementation. Instead you will end up not finishing the mini-projects that will help you accomplish your weekly weight loss goals.

In order to lose weight relentlessly, you have to consistently remind yourself to take productive action and stop allowing distractions like negative thinking and purposeless action take away your focus and keep you from achieving your daily weight-loss goals. Say "No", to the urge to eat ice cream, to try a salty delight or to simply eat more cake. Eat them when they fit into your plans and

© Dr. Chio Ugochukwu 2019-All rights reserved

not simply because others will feel bad or think you are different because you refused.

When you have realistic strategies for weight loss, taking specific steps to accomplish your goals become easier. This will help you to focus on what you can do to make things positive rather than worrying about failures and outcomes when setbacks or unexpected events happen in your life. It is being part of the solution rather than the cause. **Taking action on your positive thoughts is essential to relentless weight loss.**

Your potential is unlimited and you can achieve anything you set your mind to. As you strive to fearlessly lose weight, you will discover that there will be additional distractions and challenges. You have to be aware of the different distractions and attractions that occur during the holiday season. Birthday parties, graduation ceremonies,

© Dr. Chio Ugochukwu 2019-All rights reserved

weddings, holidays and anniversaries occur and may disrupt your well-crafted weight loss plans unless you take proactive action. Do you have a plan for celebrations? Do you snack with fruits before parties so that you won't overeat and blow up weight loss plan at the party? Do you watch what you drink? Do you reassess your focus every 15 minutes? Are you wasting time or are accomplishing your set mini-goals for the day?

The relentless weight loss program requires consistent vigilance and action. Stay focused. You can use the compass "VAM" method to make changes to your daily meals and eating habit so that you can easily achieve your specific and realistic weight loss goals in the time-frame of your choice including your Christmas party!.

© Dr. Chio Ugochukwu 2019-All rights reserved

Use the compass "VAM" method to manage your daily meals and lose weight before your Christmas party.

Do you know how you can use the compass "VAM" method to achieve your specific weight loss goals? Do you have the discipline to do easy activities daily? You can easily build up your confidence in your ability to consistently lose weight through **the compass "VAM" method for relentless weight loss** that is based on **variety, adjustments and moderation**. The order in which you make the modifications is entirely up to you. My suggestion is that you start with moderation.

The first step towards implementing your compass "VAM" method for losing weight before your Christmas party would be to cut down the servings or portions of your regular

© Dr. Chio Ugochukwu 2019-All rights reserved

meal by half. This will reduce your energy intake by about half or a third. You fill the gap with vegetables and fruits. If you feel pangs of hunger, snack with almond nuts, drink plenty of water or eat some fruits or chew some celery. When you chew celery before you go yo a party, you won't eat much because the fiber n celery will make you fill full even before you begin to eat.

Why is the reduction in portions so important? According to surveys by doctors and nutritionists the average American male takes about 3,000 calories per day and the female 2,400 calories per day (Reuters Health, 2015). According to Dr. Wang an energy intake and expenditure expert, consistent loss or reduction in energy intake of 100 calories would lead to 10 pounds loss in weight (Reuters Health, 2015). **This will happen if you make the decision to consistently reduce your**

© Dr. Chio Ugochukwu 2019-All rights reserved

daily food portion. It won't happen if you cut down your food portion in the morning then make up for it by double your usual portion in the afternoon

The more you reduce your servings, the more weight you would lose because the fewer calories you will take in, the less excess calories you will have to store as fat. However, reduced servings may mean more hunger pangs. This is a serious potential problem that could make you drink a lot of soda or eat many hot dogs as an immediate way of dealing with your hunger pangs. Unless you make adjustments this could simply lead you to more energy intake and more weight gain.

The next step in the compass "VAM" method is to make adjustments. Adjustments are changes you make to eating pattern and your meals so that you

© Dr. Chio Ugochukwu 2019-All rights reserved

can continue to lose weight and keep it off. Drinking more soda is the wrong **adjustment** for hunger pangs from portion reduction. Snacking with cookies and candies won't work. Saying , "Yes" to every offer to snack at work or at social gatherings will not help you lose weight. You have to make discipline part of your weight loss journey f you truly want lose weight before your Christmas party. The right **adjustment** would be to eat more fruits, vegetables and fibers as fillers. Fibers are especially good for your system because they help to increase bowel movement. This has the added effect of making your digestive system more efficient.

For different cultures and settings, different modifications to familiar eating habits can be made. In the United States this would entail cutting down on fast foods, soda and other

© Dr. Chio Ugochukwu 2019-All rights reserved

processed foods. According to the CDC sugar-sweetened beverages (SSBs) or sugary drinks like sodas are leading sources of added sugars in the American diet. Drinking soda is associated with weight gain/obesity, type 2 diabetes, gout, tooth decay, heart disease, kidney diseases, and liver disease (CDC, 2017). If you want to lose weight before your Christmas party you have to stop drinking sugar-sweetened beverages like soda, fruit-juice and fruit punch. **Drink water or unsweetened tea instead of soda. Add chia seeds to a cup of yoghurt and make it your snack. It will you to eat away excessive weight fast!**

Another adjustment could be to stop eating processed food like bread. Did you know that bread can be a source of sodium and too much energy intake? Did you know that on the average a slide of bread contains 150 mg of sodium and 110

© Dr. Chio Ugochukwu 2019-All rights reserved

calories per serving? This would mean that for bread with one slice per serving, 10 slices would be 1100calories. This would be more than half of the average 2000 calories per day recommended for most people.

The second reason may be related to your snacking habits. Did you know that one small pack of unsalted peanuts contained 220 calories per serving but 6 servings per pack? How does this information which you read from the nutrition facts on the pack help you? It can help you determine calories per pack, sodium per pack and sugar per pack

.

Be careful with snacks!!! Did you know that when you finish a pack of peanuts rich in dietary fiber, with little or zero sodium and cholesterol, you are also eating more than more 1000 calories. When you combine it with 1100 calories from 10 slices

© Dr. Chio Ugochukwu 2019-All rights reserved

of bread or even ice cream, you can see why your weight loss strategy may fail. This shows that you also have to pay attention to the size and frequency of your snacks if you want to quickly lose weight.

If you want to lose weight and keep it off, you have to know your daily sources of extra calories. Do you know how many calories you have in your morning cereal or pack of pea nuts? When you regularly read the nutritional facts in the food you eat, you can find out calories per serving. This is part of the adjustment part of the compass "VAM" strategy for weight loss before your Christmas party.

Apart from the adjustments I have mentioned so far, another easy one, you can quickly do, is to start drinking a glass of water before each meal.

© Dr. Chio Ugochukwu 2019-All rights reserved

This will make feel full, without eating as much as before. After a while, you will be able to consistently cut down on your daily portions of food or snacks.

Research has shown that drinking water before a meal will help to expand your stomach. This approach will make you feel completely full when you are only 80% full. This is important because eating only up to 80 % full was one of the common practices of people of Okinawa in Japan, who have the highest number of centenarians in the world (Boyle & Long, 2010).

If you want to easily lose weight before your Christmas party then drink at least two glasses of water per meal and increase the bulk in your meals through fruits and vegetables. **This will help you**

© Dr. Chio Ugochukwu 2019-All rights reserved

reduce your total calorie intake per meal without tortures diets.

To increase your intake of fruits and vegetables, start by eating every meal with salads consisting of cabbage, tomatoes, carrots, broccoli, spinach and bananas. Eating a colorful variety of fruits and vegetables per meal with reduced portions of brown rice will make your meal significantly more healthy and more bulky but less energy dense. It will help you to lose significant pounds and keep them off. **Remember calories in calories out.**

Also remember that the **Compass "VAM" Method is based on variety, adjustments and moderation (VAM). To make sustainable adjustments and modifications to your meals concentrate on variety and moderation.** Include chicken, fish, beans, cottage cheese, chia seeds or

© Dr. Chio Ugochukwu 2019-All rights reserved

low fat yogurt in your meals. You can make low fat yogurt and chia seed for your snack or even breakfast. Have eggs, nuts and red meat occasionally. You can further reduce your fat intake by eating skinless chicken or turkey. Turkey and chicken have their fat on their skin but red meat has most of its fat contained within the meat. Grilling is better than frying, and always aim to use unsaturated oils like corn, and olive oils for cooking.

You can also gradually reduce the fat content in your milk products. You can do this by changing the variety of milk that you drink from whole milk, to 2% fat; then to 1% fat. I am wary of fat free milk because it is still important to get fat in your body which can be used through cellular metabolism to produce cell membranes and hormones.

© Dr. Chio Ugochukwu 2019-All rights reserved

Remember that variety is the spice of life. It is the "V" in the compass "VAM" method. Do not eat the same meal day in day out. Why? It gets boring after a while and you will soon find yourself looking less excited about eating healthy. You have to like and enjoy what you eat. **Weight loss is not punishment!**

To sustainably lose weight, you have to aim for a healthy variety of food that contains adequate but moderate portions of fat, proteins, carbohydrates and vitamins that you actually like.. If you feel hungry between meals, snack with small portions of almonds, cashew nuts or peanuts. Almonds will make you feel less hungry and still boost your metabolism, though they take getting used. Have you tried almonds before? Please share your thoughts in the compass club.

© Dr. Chio Ugochukwu 2019-All rights reserved

If you plan your meals and snacks ahead of time you will have to make them the variety that will help you to relentlessly lose weight. Take time to plan at least one lunch and dinner every week without meat or cheese. Create your meals around whole grains, vegetables and beans to increase fiber and reduce fat. If you want to have something to chew on, get some fish or tofu. or pieces of celery You can make every Friday your fish meal day to begin with then gradually add more and more fish to your meals.

Have at least five servings of fruit every day. Choose fruit that is in season. Take an apple per meal. The red delicious apples contain pectin, a fiber that helps to promote healthy cholesterol levels and contain more amounts of antioxidants than many other types of apples.

© Dr. Chio Ugochukwu 2019-All rights reserved

You now have a deeper understanding of yourself in terms of holistic weight loss, a specific and realistic weight loss goal and the compass "VAM" method to help you get the results you desire quickly. However, all the depth of knowledge and insight into losing weight and keep it off, will fail unless you take action everyday!!!

© Dr. Chio Ugochukwu 2019-All rights reserved

© Dr. Chio Ugochukwu 2019-All rights reserved

Take action every day

You have to decide to do something every day that will help you lose weight. Having achievable goals and realistic strategies will not help you lose weight unless you take action every day. If you really want to relentlessly   lose weight and fulfill your daily goals and live the lifestyle of your dreams, you have to stop assuming you will do things later.

Take action now! When you have a good idea, act on it immediately with whatever resources you have at hand. Delaying taking action will lead to unintended consequences. Take action now instead of assuming you will act later.

Stop pointing fingers at others whenever things do not go as planned or you fail to do the things

© Dr. Chio Ugochukwu 2019-All rights reserved

you should have done to help you lose weight.. After all, we all make mistakes. We all have room for improvement. If you focus on taking small but productive steps every day, without allowing yourself to be bogged down by daily frustrations, challenges and criticisms you will gradually turn your life around and make it the amazing life you have always wanted it to be. Stop waiting for things to be perfect, act with what you have.

Take a deep breath and re-focus on the positive actions that can lead to the results you want. Look at the patterns or circumstances that usually lead to anxieties and troublesome behaviors that stop you from taking action every day. Try as much as possible to modify these patterns every day. This will help you avoid behavior that drains your energy and wastes your time. Time is a limited commodity so it has to be used wisely. **"Yesterday" used to be "Tomorrow".** Assuming

© Dr. Chio Ugochukwu 2019-All rights reserved

you will do things later is one way of mismanaging time and making your gain weight daily instead of losing it.

Identify situations and events that make it difficult for you to get the results you want from your behavior. If everyone in your office is always urging you to eat food that you do not consider healthy, what will you do? Will you cave in? Will you refuse and or explain why you have to stick to your guns now? The more you can consistently take action everyday, the more you can consistently lose weight daily. Do not wait for the perfect preparation. Stop assuming you will start later because you may never start at all.

You cannot relentlessly lose weight daily and throughout the year if your days are dotted with unfinished or and uncompleted projects. Did you not know that not having a reliable and consistent

© Dr. Chio Ugochukwu 2019-All rights reserved

approach to weight –loss can lead a pursuit of too many strategies with more anxiety, more stress and potentially more errors? Do you know that when you are distracted by lack of time, you end up rushing through your tasks without giving them the thorough attention they would require to produce great results?

This would include rushing through your food, your exercise routine and your communication strategies for dealing with unexpected challenges and setbacks. Trust the individualized process you have developed for yourself through the compass profiles and the compass "VAM" method for weight loss. Take action now!

When you begin to take daily action to lose weight, you will have successes and challenges. If you find yourself discouraged by what others might say or do, make an effort to communicate

© Dr. Chio Ugochukwu 2019-All rights reserved

positively with yourself. If you don't, the negative comments and words of discouragement from others will challenge your ability to stay the course. Make your communication strategies part of your daily activities to help you lose weight and keep it off.

© Dr. Chio Ugochukwu 2019-All rights reserved

© Dr. Chio Ugochukwu 2019-All rights reserved

Use effective communication strategies to help you quickly lose weight before your Christmas party

Did you know that communication is an important part of weight loss? Do you remember that the "C" in the compass profiles represents community relationships and communications? You can use your communication strategy to foresee and rule your daily encounters with others. If you are dealing with a difficult person or someone who is usually quick to judge or very negative in outlook be prepared to bend without breaking. Remember that most things in life are transitional, including such conversations. Don't let such negative conversations derail you from your goal of sustainable weight loss.

© Dr. Chio Ugochukwu 2019-All rights reserved

If you want to remain on track with your weight loss program throughout your daily interactions every day, you have to be able to recognize hidden antagonistic conversational messages and deal with them. Your inner voice can make a huge difference in your focus, success and ability to lose weight quickly day by day.

After you have gained a deeper understanding of why you're bombarding yourself with negative thoughts you can use effective communication strategies to anticipate what you might say to yourself during certain situations and "rewrite" the dialogue. You can use effective communication strategies to encourage yourself to keep on trying to lose weight and keep it off, even when other factors like your job, social role, family dynamics and daily encounters with others push you in the opposite direction. If the dialogue doesn't quite go

© Dr. Chio Ugochukwu 2019-All rights reserved

the way you planned it in your mind, you can do this through the EFRAMES communication strategy.

If you don't know about EFRAMES, read my book, "9 ways to keep stress out your relationships…" to get more details. In EFRAMES, "E" stands for "emphasizing empathy throughout your interactions with others". "F" stands for "find and focus on the facts", and "R" for read body language. "A" is for assessing relationship interactions. The remaining elements of the EFRAMES framework are "MES". M stands for maintain self-esteem in your interaction and relationships. "E" stands for evaluate everything in your interaction with others. **The elephant always looks different for everyone**. "S" stands for summarize your interactions through self–assertiveness while supporting your

© Dr. Chio Ugochukwu 2019-All rights reserved

position with facts and being mindful of the other person's feelings.

When it comes to daily communications, it is important to pay particular attention to how you relate to your family, friends and.co-workers. Though your family may love you and genuinely want the best for you, you still have to take daily action to get the best out of your life. This is because family members can be brutally critical of your efforts when the results they get out of your efforts do need meet their emotional and financial needs. Use your self-talk to prepare yourself for the unexpected. Stick to your weight loss goals even if they are not universally approved.

The bottom line is that whether you are dealing with friends, families or co-workers, it is important to make sure you understand the full meaning of

© Dr. Chio Ugochukwu 2019-All rights reserved

your conversations with them. If you are not able to do this you will find yourself constantly having misunderstandings and shouting matches with your friends and loved ones. This will lead to daily anxiety, criticisms and frustrations that can drain your energy and ultimately diminish your ability to lose weight relentlessly unless you change your thought process and make your communication more effective.

If you change your way of thinking, you will change your life and overcome the fear of failure which can stop you from trying your best to lose weight and keep it off. Learn to say "No" to people who are constantly trying to get you to try those snacks you have already told them you do not want because you are trying to lose weight. They may be your friends but they are not helping in your weight-loss journey. They are pointing you in the

© Dr. Chio Ugochukwu 2019-All rights reserved

wrong direction, and listening to them will make you fail.

Picture yourself winning in those scenarios and think deeply about how you would feel after you have successfully lost weight and kept it off. **Celebrate small victories along the way but be prepared for unexpected setbacks.** Having small victories as you pursue your ultimate dream will train you for greater success.

Not everyone will be happy to see that you have not given up on your dreams or that you refuse to let the fear of failure stop you from trying. If you stay focused and refuse to let what others think about you determine how you feel, you will eventually get most of what you want from your daily opportunities.

Don't let your day be full of missed opportunities. Learn to see the possibility for weight loss in every

© Dr. Chio Ugochukwu 2019-All rights reserved

encounter or event that makes up your day. You can do this by directing your energy into making the most out of your daily situations instead of trying to determine whom to blame or whom to chastise. Focus on taking advantage of your daily opportunities rather than on the words and actions of those who generate a lot of negative energy with little or no capacity to support your goals.

Remember that before you can take advantage of your daily opportunities you have to recognize them. You have to know when important opportunities have come your way. Do you look at your daily challenges and setbacks as opportunities to continue with your relentless weight loss program? Do you look at them as proof of your inability to succeed?

If you really want to lose weight relentlessly you have to make consistent adjustments through

© Dr. Chio Ugochukwu 2019-All rights reserved

effective communication strategies. You can do this by making sure that you make your perspectives in such a way that you stay innovative all the time. You cannot allow the fear of failure stop you from trying or prevent you from making full use of your daily opportunities. *Ozaa Akwusina* (A warrior never stops).

You have to learn to minimize the tendency to think of the worst outcomes all the time. **Rather than thinking the worst about a situation or an event, remind yourself that remaining positive through difficult times will help you to transform your daily reality. This type of focus will help you to continue to lose weight even if all those around you think that you can't.**

If you do not invest in yourself and in your ability to find out new and better ways to make the most out of your daily opportunities, your dreams and

© Dr. Chio Ugochukwu 2019-All rights reserved

goals will remain illusions to be pursued but ultimately unrealized. You can avoid such an outcome by learning how to spot opportunities and consistently take positive action to transform your opportunities into accomplishments.

You also have to learn how to communicate with yourself and others in a way that makes your relationships mutually beneficial. This will make you feel good about yourself and make you less moody and less likely to eat disruptively. Effective communication strategies are important because according to Burley-Allen (1995), words can affect our biases and lead to uncomfortable emotions and negative reactions. Unfortunately, some of these negative reactions may include giving up on the actions that can help you lose weight because of what others have said or implied. Don't give up. Refocus and evaluate your progress and challenges throughout your weight loss journey!!!

© Dr. Chio Ugochukwu 2019-All rights reserved

© Dr. Chio Ugochukwu 2019-All rights reserved

Make regular evaluation part of your weight loss strategy

Do you weigh yourself every 3days or at least once a week? Get a weight-loss journal or notebook. Unless you have a way to regularly evaluate your progress throughout your weight loss journey, you will not have concrete success. How can you tell your daily mini goals if you don't evaluate yourself? Are you regularly eating your variety of vegetables and fruits? Are you still reducing your food portions or have slowly gone back to your old portion? Do you still exercise regularly or have discovered that "you don't have time"? Are you keeping stress out of your relationships and conversations?

To lose weight relentlessly throughout the year you have be able to measure and demonstrate to

© Dr. Chio Ugochukwu 2019-All rights reserved

yourself that what you are doing is working. You have to make your daily mini-goals are subset of your main goal for the week and for the month. If you do not do this, despite your best intentions, you will end up not losing as much weight as you would like to.

After you have determined or discovered the easy activities that will consistently help you to lose weight, take realistic action to transform yourself and get the results you want for yourself. Your goals should be achievable and make sense within the parameters of your life. One way to check your progress in your weight loss journey is to take regular measurements. You can do this by weighing yourself every week, measuring your waist circumference every month and calculating your BMI every six months. You can also use less formal ways like dress size, change in belt hole, pant size, loose ring, or

© Dr. Chio Ugochukwu 2019-All rights reserved

changes in shoe fitting to evaluate your weight loss journey.

Through this book you already know the steps you need to take to help you lose   weight every day. Check your list of activities you consider realistic for you to accomplish your weight loss in a day based on your knowledge, experience, personality, available resources and your time –management skills. Once you have a concrete list in front of you, it's a lot easier to check on yourself regularly. You have to stick to your plan and accomplish the tasks on your list one after the other. If you do this day in, day out, week after week, you will easily lose weight throughout the year without gaining it back! Do you have the discipline to do your best with what you have every day?

© Dr. Chio Ugochukwu 2019-All rights reserved

© Dr. Chio Ugochukwu 2019-All rights reserved

Maintain your discipline and do your best with what you have

Do you remember exactly what you were doing at this time yesterday? Was that activity helping you in losing weight or gaining weight? Did someone make you eat too much or did you resist and eat right? Were you making the best use of your time? Everyone has 24 hours in a day. If you truly want to lose weight before your Christmas party, you have to start where you are. Can you find time to walk for five more minutes though your schedule is full? Can you do more to keep stress out of your life? Can you stick to a simple and easy weight loss plan? Are you doing the best you can,with what you have?

The key to making the best out of what you have by day by day is the discipline that will help you

© Dr. Chio Ugochukwu 2019-All rights reserved

improve every day. The "O" in the compass method stands for operational capacity profile. Without a disciplined and focused use of your time and resources your desire to quickly lose weight will fail. You have to make discipline the anchor of your daily focus. You cannot win without taking consistent action. You cannot achieve your weight loss goals without discipline.

Discipline is like the ladder of success, climbing it one step at a time will help you achieve your goals and much more. If you do not pay attention to your steps as you climb up a ladder, you may end up falling. This means that if you do not have situational awareness while eating, you may eat more than you planned and find yourself gaining weight at the same time. If you truly want to lose weight relentlessly every day you have to have the situational awareness and discipline to say "No" to friends, coworkers, and well-wishers who want

© Dr. Chio Ugochukwu 2019-All rights reserved

you to try one delightful, amazing delicious food or another!

Without discipline you cannot implement your best ideas for long enough to get the results to help you lose weight and live the lifestyle of your dreams. This means that if you have decided to walk a mile everyday then you have to follow through until you get the benefits you desire. If you have decided to read your nutrition facts before every meal, stick to it. You have decide on the minimum amount of exercise you shall do every day and do it. You have to be consistent in keeping your portions small and maintaining the variety of your food with more emphasis on fruits, vegetables and fish.

A disciplined approach to life either through regular exercise or better time management will help you manage stress better and accomplish

© Dr. Chio Ugochukwu 2019-All rights reserved

more throughout the day. This will also help you build up confidence in your ability to carry out your daily weight loss plans. Stress can be very disruptive. It can disrupt your ability to concentrate and stay focused on the task of the moment. It can have an overwhelming and detrimental effect on your lifestyle and confidence. When stress escalates, it throws your whole life out of balance, including your plan to lose weight relentlessly. Unfortunately the holiday season and Christmas period can quite stressful: the need to buy presents attend parties in your best outfits, can lead to unexpected consequences.

This imbalance can drain you physically, emotionally and mentally. It can lead to unwanted stress and may even affect your self-confidence and your ability to interact positively with others. This has the potential to lead to negative coping

© Dr. Chio Ugochukwu 2019-All rights reserved

mechanisms like resorting to emotional eating to cope with stress.

When stress leads you to a disruptive place, press the pause button. Trust the process you have already determined works best for you and begin again. Discipline and confidence in yourself will help you determine when to eat, when to watch others eat or when to simply walk away. Constant pressure can occur through your daily interactions with yourself and others.

Can you withstand the pressure when the negative comments start trickling in? Can you refuse to participate in the activities you really like so that you can focus on the activities that will help you lose weight? Can you refuse to eat "good" food that may not be good for your own health when everyone around you is asking you to do so? Will you have the discipline to refuse your favorite TV

© Dr. Chio Ugochukwu 2019-All rights reserved

shows or Netflix movie because you watching screen time can lead to unintended consequences?

Do you have the discipline to refuse to be distracted by the latest trend or latest "great idea"? When you get to the point where you can more consistently focus and achieve your daily mini-goals you will begin to develop the confidence that will help you to lose weight even when others expect you to fail.

The confidence that comes from successful repeated executions of small daily tasks is what will help you put enough trust and confidence in yourself to eliminate unnecessary doubt. Unnecessary doubt is an attribute that will make you double check and triple check your work until you end up making avoidable mistakes, rejecting good products, missing your mini-goals or losing confidence in yourself.

© Dr. Chio Ugochukwu 2019-All rights reserved

If you lack confidence in yourself and you spend your time and your life seeking approval from others before you complete your projects or try to fulfill your daily dreams and goals, you will be disappointed. You will not be able to quickly lose weight before your Christmas party, because you will unwisely spend most of your time and energy focusing on those who are either not prepared to give you the support you need or frankly lack the ability to give you that support.

Consistent confidence will help you to maintain the discipline that you will need to handle the different circumstances that you will encounter in the limited time that you have to lose weight before your Christmas party! This will help you to overcome the natural tendency to lose confidence when things are not working as you would like them to. It will also help you to pay less emphasis on the results of your efforts and more on the

© Dr. Chio Ugochukwu 2019-All rights reserved

process. **Ask yourself, right now, "Are you making the best possible use of this moment in time?"**

Do not waste your time looking for the perfect plan or start one plan and give it up and start another one? Instead of trying to get the perfect plan or looking for perfect co-workers or perfect friends, do the best you can where you are, with what you have. I know this is a mouthful!! Essentially it boils down to focusing on doing your best with what you have instead of complaining about what you do not have that you could have used to do a better job. You can do this by creating an individualized plan and a mental picture that will help you to maintain a sharp focus on your main goals by breaking them into mini-goals that you can accomplish through small but consistent daily action.

© Dr. Chio Ugochukwu 2019-All rights reserved

This is actually the key to achieving your weight – loss goals. When you are taking action that will not lead you to your designated goals for the day, you are wasting your most precious asset, time! You have to have the ability to consistently take action that will help you fulfill your goals every day. If you are not able to do this consistently you will slowly lose confidence in yourself and lack the trust in yourself to do what you have to do to lose weight before your Christmas party! Can you stay focused and refuse to quit as you continue on your weight loss journey?

© Dr. Chio Ugochukwu 2019-All rights reserved

© Dr. Chio Ugochukwu 2019-All rights reserved

Stay focused and refuse to quit even when others begin to tease you

Do you know that intention is not enough? Do you know that people will tease you and try to make fun of you, the more determined you are to lose weight? Can you stay focused on what you had in mind when you started your weight loss journey and refuse to quit? A firm goal to lose weight before your Christmas party does not mean that you will not have any failures or disappointments throughout the day. If you want to focus and thrive every day you have to have a strategic approach to daily living. Here are some strategies that will help you avoid those pitfalls that will make you fail to fulfill your daily goals.

First, focus on the positive and try to be productive everyday because negative thoughts lead to

© Dr. Chio Ugochukwu 2019-All rights reserved

negative emotions and negative outcomes. Lack of focus on the positive leads to poor management of disruptive circumstances and situations. This can to lead to frustrations, anger and less success with weight loss, unless you make adjustments. You have to remember to stay focused and refuse to quit when the going gets tough. Only relentless focus can help you accomplish your weight loss goals.

Focus on a step by step approach. First embrace the concept of holistic weight loss through a deeper understanding of your compass profile, then do your 72-hour food audit. Next use the compass "VAM, method to manage your daily meals. After you have gained a more realistic picture of how well you can manage your daily meals, this usually takes about a week or two, set realistic goals for how much weight you can lose

© Dr. Chio Ugochukwu 2019-All rights reserved

in 3 weeks and use that to decide your weight loss goal before your Christmas party.

If you plan to wear a different size dress or pants for the party, buy it. This will motivate to stay focused and the take the actions that will help you get the results that you want. Do not try to accomplish too many things in a day or you will end up getting yourself overwhelmed and disappointed with little or no time for other parts or aspects of your life.

Do not get into the habit of having too many projects up in the air at once. Finish one before you start another. Begin with end in mind also means that you have a plan for completing your projects when you start them. Don't start your projects with only the hope that you will complete them. Stay focused from the beginning to the end. Write down the day you expect to lose your first

© Dr. Chio Ugochukwu 2019-All rights reserved

10 pounds after you start. An open –ended weight loss program, discourages completion while promoting lack of focus and delays. If you truly want to transform your life and live the lifestyle of your dreams, you have to be able begin with the end in mind and stay focused on completing your projects or accomplishing your goals one step at a time.

If you truly want to consistently lose weight every day, you have to refuse to quit after you begin. Too many people begin, then quit before they get the results they desire. You have to be able to strategically put aside your daily disappointments and early failures in your attempts at losing weight. Do not let your daily struggles stop you from focusing on your specific tasks for the day. Be prepared to try your best after the disappointment of the moment or of the hour or of the day. Do you bounce back from adversity every

© Dr. Chio Ugochukwu 2019-All rights reserved

day? Do you refuse to quit? Have set up a day for fasting as part of compass VAM strategy for weight loss?

Keep in mind that difficult conditions are temporary. **Criticisms will pass if you do not keep replaying them in your mind.** Frustrations will boil over. Focus on your destinations instead of the bumps or delays along your weight loss journey. **Life is full of ups and downs. Refuse to let a rough morning spoil the rest of your day**. Don't overeat simply because no one seems to appreciate all the effort you have put into losing weight and making yourself more healthy. When things look bleak, you have to remember that you could be on the verge of a breakthrough. **Never forget that the darkest part of the night is just before dawn.**

© Dr. Chio Ugochukwu 2019-All rights reserved

Do you have a daily plan for dealing with stress? Do you eat a balanced diet, exercise regularly, and go to bed on time. Do you build the physical and mental strength to keep going when the going gets tough? **Do you bounce refuse to quit when the going gets tough. Do you stay focused?**

If you want to stay focused and refuse to quit everyday, you have to learn to stop being too harsh on yourself and learn to love yourself more everyday. Remember not to allow yourself to be distracted by trying to complete too many projects all at once. Finish one project before you start another. Learn from your mistake. Remember that the relentless weight loss program is a multifaceted process. You have to persist to win.

One of the main reasons why people fail to bounce back everyday is that they are too harsh on

© Dr. Chio Ugochukwu 2019-All rights reserved

themselves. Instead of seeing their short comings as part of the process of growth, they consider them as a confirmation that they can never be successful. You can lose as much weight as you want if you refuse to give up and continue to strive to improve. You can lose weight relentlessly if you follow your own SEPP (Strategy, Effort, Process and Persistence and TIAs (Transformational Infinite Adjustments) that will help you convert obstacles and challenges in your weight loss journey into opportunities for outstanding success. If you do this consistently every week **you will quickly lose weight that you want to lose before your Christmas party!!!**

© Dr. Chio Ugochukwu 2019-All rights reserved

© Dr. Chio Ugochukwu 2019-All rights reserved

Review and improve (RAI)

Congratulations !!! I am proud of you, for your grit and determination! **After reading this book you have to take action.** First do a one-page review in which you write down everything you have read in this book and how you will use them to lose weight before your Christmas party.

What is the essence of your compass holistic weight- loss approach? Make this your first paragraph. If you need additional help doing this, visit www.compasswellnessinstitute.com and sign up for my newsletter or simply text me, introducing yourself and asking questions on 661 992 6436.

Make a list of the barriers to your weight loss program and how you plan to overcome them

© Dr. Chio Ugochukwu 2019-All rights reserved

everyday. If you can't and need more help, please contact me for more *relentless transformational* strategies!

What is your 3-month weight loss goal? Through this compass method for weight loss and the VAM strategies , I have shared with you quickly lose 10-20 pounds in about 6 to 8 weeks.

What is your biggest challenge or area of frustration?

Slow down so that you can go faster.

Do you like the way you manage stress, time and productivity?

Don't let the perfect become the enemy of the possible.

© Dr. Chio Ugochukwu 2019-All rights reserved

Persist until success happens (PUSH).

Don't become so afraid of failing that you never begin.

How   can   you   improve?

What changes do you think you can make that will make it easier for you to lose weight before your Christmas party?

Share your thoughts and concerns by joining the compass club on Facebook so that you find out how others have tackled similar problems or challenges in their weight loss journey.

If you need one on one consultation please visit www.compasswellnessinstitute.com to sign up for the six month relentless weight loss program.

© Dr. Chio Ugochukwu 2019-All rights reserved

© Dr. Chio Ugochukwu 2019-All rights reserved

Appendix

Join the Compass Club:I1 week-Motivation Group for Weight loss To Help you lose weight before your Christmas party!

Week 1, Education and Measurements.

As you begin to apply what you have learned from this book to your circumstance and situation consider creating a group of participants that will remind each other of why losing weight is a goal for them. Each group member will have a hands on experience of how measurements like waist circumference and body mass index can used to identify whether an individual is within normal weight, overweight, or obese. For this motivation group program the definition of overweight will be based on normal (BMI<25kg/m²), overweight

© Dr. Chio Ugochukwu 2019-All rights reserved

(BMI=25-29 kg/m²), and obesity will be based on a BMI of ≥30. This was the same definition used by Koebnick et al. (2012) in their study on young adults in California. Abdominal obesity will be measured through waist circumference (WC). Severe abdominal obesity will be defined as (WC ≥ 88cm) in women and (WC ≥ 102cm) in men.

Week 2, Benefits

Each group member will write down in his weight loss journal the benefits of losing weight, which would include the reduced risk of diabetes, high blood pressure, and heart disease. Those who participate in the program will become more active and spend less time watching television. This will lead to having more time for getting work or studies done. Sleeping more hours per day and eating more healthy food would also reduce the risk of health related problems. Each group

© Dr. Chio Ugochukwu 2019-All rights reserved

member should get their weight loss journal and write down how many hours of sleep, they have every day.

Week 3, Barriers to change

Group members need to remember that the cause of obesity differs for each individual. If it is due to poor eating habits or due to poor physical activity, then it will be easier to change through eating healthy and becoming more active. However, when the cause of obesity or weight gain, includes medical illness like endocrine or neurological problems it becomes more difficult to achieve the desired change. This will require referral to the appropriate health care professional for adequate intervention.

According to Anshel (2010) sometimes the barrier to change is non-adherence to healthy habits. This is one barrier to change that can be modified by

© Dr. Chio Ugochukwu 2019-All rights reserved

self-motivation and working with group members. Encourage one another during your weekly meetings and consider doing healthy competition on weight loss. Make sure there are multiple winners in your group.

Categories can be First to lose 10 pounds

Best fruit salad

Tastiest Lunch

Least expensive fish meal

Most consistent group attendant

Easiest exercise ideas

Best jokes to deal with stress

Your group should aim to award prizes every week, for the first 11-week session of the group.

Week 4 to Week 5

Discuss a selected factor that can influence weight gain as identified through the research. Ask each

© Dr. Chio Ugochukwu 2019-All rights reserved

group member to share their own insight based on what they read about weight loss. Participants will be asked how many hours a day they spent watching television and how much they alcohol and soft drinks they drink weekly.in details per week with given goals. The goal in Week 4 will be focused on cutting down on television time to less than an hour per day, week 5 will be focused on cutting down on the drinking of alcohol and soft drinks to less than 5 times per week.

Week 6: sleep

Week 6 will be focused on increasing sleep to more than 6 hours per day. This will include discussing the role of environmental factors like extended periods of light in the room or changes in room temperature can lead to reduced hours of sleep per day (Knutson,2012). Cultural factors that

© Dr. Chio Ugochukwu 2019-All rights reserved

can influence sleep include how much value the culture or society in which one lives places on health when compared to productivity. If sleep is considered an act of laziness then most people would opt for more work hours and sleep less. Sociocultural conversations on what is normal sleep could also lead to unrealistic expectations and what constitutes normal sleep (Knutson, 2012). This could lead to anxiety and make falling asleep more difficult. Participants will be asked how many hours of sleep they have had each day and what they considered their barriers to sleeping better.

Week 7: diet moderation

Week 7 will be focused on cutting down on sweetened sugars. This is because a study by

© Dr. Chio Ugochukwu 2019-All rights reserved

Bermudez and Gao (2010) found that a greater intake of sweetened beverages was associated with a higher risk of total and abdominal obesity for young adults aged between 20-39 years of age. The study found that 10 additional teaspoons of added sugars per day were associated with a 52% higher risk of obesity. Participants will be asked how teaspoons of added sugar they consumed every day. Their goal would be to reduce the amount of added sugar they consumed every day to less than five teaspoons.

Week 8: Overcoming barriers

Week 8 will focus on increased barriers to physical activity including heightened body consciousness and a feeling of insecurity among those overweight compared to those who were not. It would also be important to allow group

© Dr. Chio Ugochukwu 2019-All rights reserved

members to discuss the role each person's ethnic background has played on how each person feels about his or her weight. This in parts of the world like the pacific Islands find being overweight is more socially acceptable and group members from such places may be less inclined to make too much effort to change or reduce their weight (Stankov, Olds, &Cargo. 2012). Participants will be asked to discuss their feelings about their weight with others and will be encouraged to increase their physical activity by walking at least 30 minutes per day. Participants will also be encouraged to discuss the influence of peer stigmatization in their lives, since research has shown that it is another factor that can prevent participation in regular physical activity

.

Week 9

© Dr. Chio Ugochukwu 2019-All rights reserved

Week 9 will focus on depressive symptoms. According to Skinner, Haines, Austin, and Field (2011) those complaining of depressive symptoms at baseline were more likely to start overeating. The prevalence of overeating increased from 2.4 % to 3.7% and the percentage of binge eating increased from 2.4% to 5.7%. The prevalence of overweight increased from 14.5% to 15.5% and obesity increased from 3% to 5.2%. Participants will be asked if they have had depressive symptoms in the past and how much they think it has affected them.

Week 10, Focus on Support

Week 10 will focus on support services. Two speakers would be invited to speak to the Participants or two participants will volunteer and do it. These two speakers will focus on helping the

© Dr. Chio Ugochukwu 2019-All rights reserved

participants determine which of the factors discussed in sessions 4 to 9 they feel is most relevant to them and share with them some of the ways they can persevere when they feel like giving up. This is important because according to Anshel (2010), 60 to 70% of adults who begin an exercise program quit in less than a year. A former group participant or someone else who has lost at least 10 pounds and kept it off for at least one year through the compass method can come and share his or her challenges, tribulations and triumphs with the group.

This type of activity prepares the way for both a short term change and a long term change. It is important to remember that obesity frequently becomes a lifelong problem. This is why everyone has to be prepared for a long term process. This will include joining support groups and making

© Dr. Chio Ugochukwu 2019-All rights reserved

changes that fit into a family's lifestyle. Friends of those trying to lose weight can help them improve their self-esteem by emphasizing their strengths and positive qualities rather than just focusing on their weight problems. The more books you read on weight loss, stress management and on personal motivation the more likely you will succeed in your own relentless weight loss program.

© Dr. Chio Ugochukwu 2019-All rights reserved

Week 11, Review

Week 11 will be a review of what has been done so far. Each participant will be given 5 minutes to share with the group what the 11-week motivation program has meant to him or her. Each participant will also be asked to say what changes they have seen in their lives as a result of their participation in the program. Participants would also be asked to say what challenges remain and what changes they will like to see in the program. Each participant will be weighed and their waist circumference measured, so that their BMI and WC can be compared to what it was at the beginning of

the program. Each participant will be given a certificate of participation and be encouraged to set monthly goals throughout the year. You can also join the compass club on

© Dr. Chio Ugochukwu 2019-All rights reserved

https://www.facebook.com/groups/1748276835431116/

for more encouragement and fun activities to help you lose weight and achieve more of your relentless transformation goals and projects.

© Dr. Chio Ugochukwu 2019-All rights reserved

© Dr. Chio Ugochukwu 2019-All rights reserved

Notes

American Heart Association (AHA).

American Academy of Child & Adolescence Psychiatry. (2011, March).*Facts for families* (Report No.79). retrieved from http:// www.aacap.org/cs/root/facts_for_families/o besity_in_children.

Anshel, M. H. (2010). The disconnected values (intervention) model for promoting healthy habits in religious institutions. *Journal of Religion and Health, 49*(1), 32-49.

Burley-Allen, M. (1995). Listening the forgotten skill: a self-teaching guide. New York, NY: John Wiley & Sons, Inc

© Dr. Chio Ugochukwu 2019-All rights reserved

Center for Disease Control and Prevention (CDC),2017

Pender, N. J., Murdaugh, C.L., & Parsons, M. A. (2011).Health promotion in nursing practice ractice.Boston:Pearson

Samaranayake, N. R., Ong, K. L., Raymond, Y.H. L.,& Chueng, B. M.Y., (2012,May). Management of obesity in the national health and nutrition examination survey (NHANES), 2007–2008. *Annals of Epidemiology, 22*(5),349-353.

Skinner, H.H. , Haines, J., Austin, S. B. , Field, A. E. (2012, May). A prospective study of overeating, binge eating, and depressive symptoms among adolescent and young adult women. *Journal of Adolescent Health, 50* (5), 478–483

Stankov, I., Olds, T., & Cargo, M. (2012). Overweight and obese adolescents: what turns

© Dr. Chio Ugochukwu 2019-All rights reserved

them off physical activity? *The International Journal of Behavioral Nutrition and Physical Activity*, *9* (1)53. Retrieved from http://www.sciencedirect.com.eaproxy.liberty.edu:2048/science/article/pii/0753332294901031

World Health Organization (WHO), 2017

© Dr. Chio Ugochukwu 2019-All rights reserved

© Dr. Chio Ugochukwu 2019-All rights reserved

Resources

Make a weight- loss journal and write a letter to yourself on how you plan to stay focused and take daily action, so that you can quickly lose weight before your Christmas party! ***Use relentless transformation to live your intended life now!!!!!!***

Here are additional resources that will help you to focus and thrive so that you can become the best and happiest version of yourself.

www.compasswellnessinstitute.com

www.compasshealthtransformer.com/members

www.dcompassmarketing.com

http://www.amazon.com/Dr.-Chio-Ugochukwu/e/B00JNFLPQQ

© Dr. Chio Ugochukwu 2019-All rights reserved

Join the compass club on Facebook

https://www.facebook.com/groups/1748276835431116/

Other books by Dr. Chio Ugochukwu that will help you get optimal health, eliminate stress, communicate better, and live your intended life include;

The Compass Health Transformer: Your 72 Hour Blue Print For Healthy Living

In this book you will learn more about how doing the 72-hour food audit can help you gain a better understanding of how you can improve your health through easy daily adjustments …..

© Dr. Chio Ugochukwu 2019-All rights reserved

21 Ways To Transform Your Health Without Medications

"…21 simple proven ways to reduce stress and improve your health and wellbeing without relying on medications. These are easy and effective ways you can use to turn your daily challenges into transformative opportunities for healthy living and daily happiness. You can start right away without spending a fortune!.."

Get your own copy of 21 Ways To Transform Your Health Without Medications

Overcoming Daily Stress: 21 Quick And Easy Ways To Stay Stress-Free In Your Daily Life

"…Are you tired of being stressed out everyday? Are you tired of feeling exhausted and overwhelmed in your daily activities? Are you fed up with communication issues in your

© Dr. Chio Ugochukwu 2019-All rights reserved

relationship? Here are 21 quick and easy ways you can use to overcome daily stress and turn your daily challenges into opportunities for transformative abundant living. This book will help you gain a better understanding of your potential communication issues, daily 'stress points' and the steps you can take to overcome them…".

Get your own copy of Overcoming Daily Stress

The Secret To Daily happiness

"..Have you ever wondered why daily happiness has continued to elude you? Do you want to make sustainable daily happiness part of your life? By reading this book you can find answers to these questions and many more on how to overcome the many obstacles and challenges that daily try to take away your inner peace and contentment…"

© Dr. Chio Ugochukwu 2019-All rights reserved

Get your own copy of The Secret To Happiness

15 Simple Ways to lower your blood pressure naturally after 40 without complicated diets

"……Don't spend your most productive years dealing with high blood pressure, medications and side effects. Stop worrying about whether you forgot to take your first medication or the second one. Take these simple steps to lower your blood pressure naturally and minimize your need for multiple medications. Did you know that high blood pressure can cause heart attack, stroke, kidney failure, blindness and memory problems? Don't wait to find out! Take Action! ,,,,,"

Click Here for Your own copy of 15 Simple Ways To Reduce Blood Pressure....

© Dr. Chio Ugochukwu 2019-All rights reserved

Here is a book to help lose fat. If your main concern or focus is losing pounds you have accumulated as fat then get a copy of the book

"How To Lose 23 Pounds of Fat Without Torture Diets or Hard Exercise And keep it (The Compass Method).

"Are you fed up with trying to lose weight again and again with limited success? Are you tired of all the confusing new and expensive diets you have tried to follow every day with zero results? Do you want the health benefits of living with optimum weight without following complicated rules? Do you want to become more energetic and active again? Are you fed up with the wild ride of losing weight today and gaining it back tomorrow? Then read this book so that you will start using a comprehensive individualized weight loss strategy that will help you lose fat and

© Dr. Chio Ugochukwu 2019-All rights reserved

keep it off, without going on torture diets or deadly strenuous exercises. You will learn to do this through the Compass Method that is based on a holistic approach to weight-loss, healthy living and personal transformation."

If prayer is something that appeals to you, you might be interested in the following next two books that incorporate prayers into our daily strive to become better and become more fulfilled:

Praying To Win: How To Get More Victories And Riches In Your Daily Life Through Spiritual Principles

"..You too can achieve your goals and dreams, through praying to win. You can do this by immersing yourself in the word of God and transforming the moments that make up your daily life through persistent adoration……. Above all,

© Dr. Chio Ugochukwu 2019-All rights reserved

thank God every day, never give up and persistently continue praying to win…"

Get your own copy of Praying To Win

9 Best Ways To Eliminate Stress, Improve Your Health And thrive Without Limitations Through Prayers

Are tired of being knocked down by stress from your daily hassles? Are you tired of dealing with chronic illnesses associated with stress? Do you want to live a fun-filled daily life? Here are 9 of the best ways you can change your daily obstacles and challenges into opportunities to thrive without limitations through the power of prayers.

Too Young To Die

"A book about coping with grief and finding your way in life…"

© Dr. Chio Ugochukwu 2019-All rights reserved

9 Best Ways To Quit Smoking Without Becoming A Nervous Wreck And Gaining Weight

"..Here are 9 of the best ways to finally quit smoking without becoming a nervous wreck or gaining weight. If you have tried to quit smoking before, but failed or tried to quit but was overcome by anxiety or fear of becoming socially awkward or gaining weight, then read this book! This book was previously published as "The Compass Health Transformer Quit Smoking", but has been rewritten to include the transtheoretical model of change to help you get a better understanding of where you are in your journey or process of quitting smoking. The 9 best ways to quit smoking also includes a reminder of the different ways smoking can affect your health and body and the different individualized-changes you can make to

© Dr. Chio Ugochukwu 2019-All rights reserved

your life-style to help you quit smoking on your own terms.

9 Best Ways To Deal With Negative People, Protect Your Health And Be Happy

"..Are you tired of being stressed out by encounters with negative people? Are you fed up with the impact of negative situations on your health and happiness? Would like you to find out ways to remain effective during negative situations and encounters with negative people? Do you know that chronic stress generated by negative encounters can damage your eyes, heart and brain? Do you know that chronic stress can directly damage your body cells? Here are 9 best ways you can protect your health from such negative situations so that you can continue to thrive and be happy..".

Are You Tough Enough To Be Great?

© Dr. Chio Ugochukwu 2019-All rights reserved

"..Have you discovered what you really want in life? Have you discovered why you were born? Do you know the direction you are going with your life….Learn more about how you can use the growth mindset to help you strive to excel in everything that you do in spite of distractions and challenges….You will discover more strategies that will help you seek excellence in everything that you do so that **you can become unstoppable and live unlimited! BULU!! Become Unstoppable, Live Unlimited. BULU!!!**

To order new or additional copies or ask questions, please visit:

http://www.amazon.com/Dr.-Chio-Ugochukwu/e/B00JNFLPQQ

Call or Text : 661 992 6436

© Dr. Chio Ugochukwu 2019-All rights reserved

You can also get courses on wellness and transformational living from

www.compasswellnessinstitute.com/courses

Join the Compass club @

https://www.facebook.com/compassclub

© Dr. Chio Ugochukwu 2019-All rights reserved

About the Author

Dr. Chio Ugochukwu has always been interested in helping people improve their health, eliminate stress, and develop the communication and leadership skills that would enable them to live their intended lives despite their busy schedules, daily challenges and duties.

He was inspired to develop **The Compass Program for optimal health, effective communication, and transformational leadership**, through the challenges he has encountered in his journey of life, his practice of medicine, his heritage of the ancient Ozaa Akwusina code and hisfascination with how the mind, the spirit, human experience, and relentless

© Dr. Chio Ugochukwu 2019-All rights reserved

transformation, influence your ability to live your intended life.

You can sign up for the Compass Program at www.compasswellnessinstitute.com.

or dcompassmarketing.com

Dr. Chio Ugochukwu is the medical director of Dala Compass Foundation and a Toastmasters International competent communicator (CC) and competent Leader (CL). He is also a bestselling author with more than 30 books on optimal health, motivation, stress elimination, weight loss, and transformative living with peer-reviewed publications on quality of life and numerous articles on stress, effective communication, healthy living and relentless transformation. He is also a healthcare and health systems consultant with the Compass Consultants International (CCI).

© Dr. Chio Ugochukwu 2019-All rights reserved

© Dr. Chio Ugochukwu 2019-All rights reserved

www.ingramcontent.com/pod-product-compliance
Lightning Source LLC
Chambersburg PA
CBHW070427290526
45791CB00005B/1872